I0429588

HEALTH MYTHS & FACTS.

GET IT RIGHT!

DR. AUGUSTA McANGUS.

CONTENTS

DEDICATION

▶ To God Almighty, for the book writing inspiration and calling into the ministry of gathering souls for Him through healthcare.

ACKNOWLEDGEMENT

▸ My heartfelt gratitude goes to:

▸ My mother, for her prayers and love.

▸ To my loving husband, my editor-in-chief who inspirited the first compilation.

▸ To Olusegun Japhet Ojo and few diamante (2007 class of Medicine & Dentistry) of my great alumni, University of Benin.

▸ And for everyone who will read this write up and make good use of it by propagating the right facts including YOU.

▸ May God reward you all, Amen.

PREFACE

▶ Health myths and facts, is a collection of superstitious beliefs across the globe, especially Nigeria.

▶ It is hoped that readers will have basic understanding in dispersing the true positions in health practice.

▶ Remember, "practice makes perfect", thus, we learn best by practicing and teaching the right position, correctly.

▶   GET IT RIGHT!

INTRODUCTION – DEFINITION AND EFFECTS OF MYTHS.

▸ Myths are false, unverifiable, common, local perceptions and popular beliefs.

▸ Myths and superstitions are borne out of real life experience-["red herring"/mistakes] and seen by many as, scientific hypothesis needing proofs.

▸ We live in a community where medical problems are deep rooted in the belief system of the people.

▸ Medical myths and misconceptions contribute to incorrect health seeking response and treatments.

▸ Mostly propagated by the non-lettered and those having minimal or no contact with skilled health workers.

▶ Some tend to use what worked for someone else forgetting the "individualized approach" to health.

▶ This makes it difficult to seek doctor's opinion but choose other family members' or neighbour's opinions. This also dictates their choice of traditional treatment over orthodox.

▶ These misconceptions will be considered along with the credible positions in series, ranging from reproductive health, maternal and child health, nutritional health to geriatrics;

EXAMPLES OF VARIOUS MYTHS AND THE CREDIBLE POSITIONS.

▶ Myth#1: Catching toilet infection from a public toilet!

▶ Truth#1: There is no infection called "toilet infection". Chances of catching any disease except cold from the toilet, is nearly zero. You cannot catch STD from a toilet seat, but only from direct sexual contact, blood transmission or from mother to her unborn child.

▶ The so-called toilet infection is a misnomer for mostly vaginal thrush also known as candidiasis. It could also be Urinary Tract Infection. People with Sexually Transmitted Infections from multiple sexual partners commonly use it as cover up.

▶ To prevent this so-called toilet infection, ensure clean, moderate and loose cotton under wears, avoid washing or douching the vagina with antiseptics and medicated soaps and liquids like dettol, without medical indication or prescription, avoid multiple sex partners and treat both partners promptly.

▶ Ensure good toilet hygiene – cleaning up from vagina to anus and not the other way round.

▶ Avoid visibly dirty toilets, wash your hands after use and take common sense precautions. There is no need to avoid public bathrooms for fear of catching "toilet infection", when nature calls.

▶ Myth #2: "MALARIA & TYPHOID SYNDROME". Most Nigerians consider and treat any febrile illness as "malaria & typhoid", because test result revealed, parasite was seen in blood film and titre for widal test is significant.

▶ No thanks to the fact that in Nigeria, it is the norm for anyone to walk into a laboratory to order or request investigations, and go to pharmacy for drugs without having to give detailed health history or be physically examined by a medical doctor.

▸ Truth #2: Widal test is not gold standard test for typhoid. Titre concentration is almost always high in severe malaria and other febrile illnesses. Yes, we live in a malaria endemic zone but It is not compulsory malaria and typhoid co-infect.

▸ Check and keep the record of your titre value when not ill for reference purposes to avoid false positive and negative values. Do blood culture and/or stool mcs to confirm. Better still, see a doctor and help save Nigeria from impending antibiotics resistance!

▸ Myth#3: Drinking mixtures like alabukun powder and schweppes bitter lemon drink with post coital exercise and washing up as a form of contraceptive method.

▶ Truth#3: Post coital exercise and washing up is ineffective as a form of contraceptive method. Visit the Family planning clinic and get informed. Not all methods stop you from having more babies when you want to.

▶ Myth#4: Vaginal douching prevents infections.

▶ Truth#4: Vaginal douching-is an unnecessary and harmful practice which in the "author's" opinion is a form of masturbation. Vaginal is a self cleaning organ. One has no business washing and stroking everyday with soap or any other douching agent. Good Toilet hygiene know-how is the way forward.

▶ Myth#5: Sperm that flow out of vagina hours after sex is "watery" and is a cause of infertility.

▶ Truth#5: It is normal for sperm to liquefy and flow out, "watery" hour(s) after sex especially on getting up from sleeping/ lying position. If in doubt of sperm quality, send for laboratory analysis. No room for guess work.

▶ Myth#6: Uterine fibroids eat up babies

▶ Truth#6: Uterine fibroids do not eat up babies in the womb and does not ALWAYS cause infertility in women. Its location and size may determine the severity of menstrual cramps and amount of blood loss during menstruation, ability to carry pregnancy to term or have vaginal delivery, etc.

▶ Myth#7: Blood tonic use is necessary while using antibiotics and antimalarials.

▶ Truth#7: The mechanism of action of antimalarial includes haemolysing red blood cells. This is not applicable for all antibiotics. Even in the face of haemolysis, the author is of the school of thought that, parasite may compete with the body system for it & blood capsules and tonics are unnecessary until after course of treatment of antimalarial for replacement, and if need be.

▶ Myth#8: Give multivitamins to EVERY child not eating well.

▶ Truth#8: There are various reasons why a toddler or child will refuse food. Giving multivitamins to boost their appetite is wickedness in instances like sore throat from tonsilitis, adenoidal enlargement among other childhood diseases, a child dependent on being spoon fed, and undiagnosed sickle cell disease especially when it contains iron, a contra-indication for use.

▶ Myths#9: Epilepsy is contagious through saliva of the affected person and primarily occurs in a person who the occult people have invoked lizard upon, to disturb their body system.

▶ Truth#9: Epilepsy is a neurological disease that can be managed with medications and rarely, surgery. It is NOT spread by contact with saliva, sharing utensils or making jest of person with epilepsy.

▶ Myth#10: Tooth eruption in children, "teething" causes fever, diarrhoea, vomiting, weight loss, cough, etc

▶ Truth#10: Apart from mild itching and/or pains, teething in normal children, tooth eruption does not cause any systemic illness or cluster of symptoms like fever, vomiting, cough etc. Poor hygiene is responsible for most of the clusters of symptoms. It may coincide with other childhood illnesses.

▶ Teething medications especially powders, contains mainly pcm and promethazine/piriton causing drowsiness.

▶ Ensure good hygiene concerning toys and other stuffs, babies use to scratch gums. Diarrhea from poor hygiene should not be treated as teething problems.

▶ Myth#11: Malformed babies occur as a result of the personality who walked across your legs while lying or sitting or the mere sighting of a masquerade/ corpse/ midget/ pygmy / Gremlin hybrid, especially during pregnancy.

▶ Truth #11: Most malformations occur during the age of viability from drug use or infections that cross the placenta.

▶ Myth#12: Increased frequency of sex reduces the risk of prostate cancer in men.

▶ Truth#12:Frequent ejaculations (>21 monthly), whether through intercourse, wet dreams/nocturnal emission, or masturbation, decreases a man's risk for prostate cancer but does not translate into license for multiple sexual partners.

▶ Myth#13: Original product is always expensive.

▶ Truth#13: High/Increased cost does not guarantee quality/effectiveness if all other things being equal and assuming it is not fake, expired, repackaged or substandard.

▶ Myth#14: Cold water is not good for children.

▶ Truth#14: Cold water does no harm to any normal and healthy child or adult. It may be limited, but not to be totally avoided when a child is ill or has cough.

▶ Myth#15: Only hopeless cases are referred.

▶ Truth#15: Referral to a higher hospital is not a death sentence. It is actually supposed to provide best chance of survival for patient. There are various reasons for referral ranging from no bed space to non-availability of best specialized personnel for the index case.

▶ Myth#16: Eating late at night does not cause weight gain.

▶ Truth#16: It is not when you eat, but how and what you eat.

▶ Myth#17: Blood shot eyes in newborns is caused by maternal posture or bending during pregnancy.

▶ Truth#17: Blood shot eyes in newborns are mostly caused by trauma to the eye during vaginal examination in labour.

▶ Myth#18: Real women deliver per vagina.

▶ Truth#18: Vaginal birth should not be a determinant for what "dignifies" womanhood. Not everybody will deliver Per Vagina. Assisted deliveries like CS are heavenly ordained and were used by the "non-Hebrew" women in bible days though undocumented.

▶ Do not attempt Vaginal Delivery after 2CS. Do not tempt God. Ensure a supervised delivery after 1CS.

▶ Myth#19: Skip breakfast when you are watching your weight.

▶ Truth#19: Breakfast is a necessary meal of the day. Never skip especially if you are watching your weight. It causes more harm than good.

▶ Myth#20: Menses is necessary to cleanse/clear the system. Trouble for menopausal women.

▶ Truth#20: Menses doesn't cleanse/clear the system. It is safe and healthy for Family Planning methods to cause amenorrhea. Menses is blood loss from a "regretful/crying" non-pregnant uterus.

▶ Menopausal women, please feel free to enjoy your sex life. Sperm will not accumulate dirt/waste in the womb or body.

▶ Myth#21: Mixture of tomato paste and malt can replace blood instead of blood transfusion.

▶ Truth#21: Blood loss at child birth or menstruation known as menorrhagia cannot be replaced with tomato-paste. Immediate replacement by blood transfusion but gradual replacement by iron tablets, fresh vegetables, fortified malt and milk.

▶ Myths#22: Taking cold drinks during pueperium causes "bad blood" storage in the body system.

▶ Truth#22: Allow women in pueperium to take desired food and cold drinks. It doesn't clog/clot blood in the womb. Hot water drinking and punching is unnecessary punishment.

▶ Myth#23: Bending over during pueperium cause pueperal psychosis by "blood rushing into the brain".

▶ Truth#23: Pueperal psychosis is of psycho-traumatic origin and never a result of posture.

▶ Myth#24: Urine is dark because of malaria.

▶ Truth#24: Dark coloured urine is not always a result of malaria. Other causes include: dehydration, diet, drugs, other hemolytic diseases.

▶ Myth#25: After exposure to sunlight, wash your breast with cold water before feeding baby.

▶ Truth#25: Unexpressed Breast milk is always at body temperature. It is unnecessary to wash breast from sunlight exposure before feeding a child. It will not cause stomach ache or harm the baby in any way.

▶ Myth#26: Tooth removal in sequence.

▶ Truth#26: Tooth pains are not caused by worms. Removal of one tooth does not lead to removal of another. Regular dental check up: S&P 6mthly, flossing, twice daily brushing, balanced nutrition especially dairy food is advised for strong teeth.

▶ Myth#27: Sugarcane water and/or Beecham Ampiclox always cure Jaundice in newborn.

▶ Truth#27: Ampiclox does not prevent or cure all forms of jaundice. All jaundice case must be assessed by health worker +/- Serum bilirubin estimation.

▶ Single dose by Beecham will do nothing. Remember cost does not guarantee quality.

▶ Treating jaundice with glucose water, sugar cane extract etc is useless EXCEPT its hunger related.

▶ Myth#28: Sex in the afternoon produce albino babies.

▶ Truth#28: genetics play a great role in this. Afternoon sex is not the reason for producing albino babies.

▶ Myth#29: Stop all diarrhoea with flagyl.

▶ Truth#29: Flagyl, aka metronidazole use for all forms of diarrhoea is drug abuse. ORS and Zn tablets best treatment for diarrhoea. If persist, ensure proper toilet hygiene, do m/c/s and see a doctor.

▶ Myth#30: White thread stops hiccups.

▶ Truth#30: White threads on newborn head can not stop hiccups. It basically stops on its own, white thread or not.

▶ Myth#31: Fan and AC causes pneumonia.

▶ Truth#31: AC / Fans do not worsen or predispose to pneumonia. Excessive dressing will not prevent it either, instead irritability from heat rash manifesting as excessive cry, excessive sweating will lead to weight loss, "Failure to Thrive" or grow in babies.

▶ Clean fan blades, AC vents and environment. Cough and catarrh should be monitored before it progresses to pneumonia.

▶ Colds are caused by hundreds of microorganisms especially viruses. They are spread by direct contact with other infected people through sharing personal belongings, sneeze, handshake, kiss etc. Yes, cold is more likely to spread during harmattan/ dry season, but being exposed to cold weather does not necessarily cause them.

▶ Myths#32: Once you stop breastfeeding, don't recommence.

▶ Truth#32: Recommencement / Resumption of breastfeeding after even more than 1-4 weeks break will not make the breast milk sour nor cause diarrhea / purge the child, as long as the mother is alive. Nowadays, breast milk is now being sold even online in the western world.

▶ Myth#33: No sugar to children's food because it makes them hyper.

▶ Truth#33: Adding moderate amount of sugar to sweeten feeds for children will not really make the child hyperactive or purge. Limiting sugar in children though can help prevent obesity, tooth decay/cavities, and loss of appetite for healthy foods. Before you feed the child, ask yourself if you can eat all of the food prepared for the child, in that state?

▶ Sugar-laden cakes, lollies and soft drinks at birthday parties should be allowed once in a while.

▶ Watch out for lactose intolerance though. Some food additives may contain aspartame in quantities that could be harmful to some children.

▶ Myth#34: Applying concoction to "dividing" anterior and posterior fontanelles.

▶ Truth#34: Ant. & post. Fontanelles are normal openings in ALL children that fuse at 18-24mths & 3mths respectively. If depressed, consider dehydration from poor feeding, diarrhoea and vomiting, excessive sweating etc. it should not be tensed or bulging either. If in doubt, see a doctor.

▶ Applying concoction disturbs head circumference growth/expansion.

▶ Myths#35: Breast milk is not satisfying enough for newborns. Hence need for supplements.

▶ Truth#35: Breastfeed newborns if possible, at least every 3-4hrs over 15-30mins and not three times a day like adult, before concluding it is not satisfying the baby.

▶ Substitute when introduced after 4-6mths should be constituted correctly.

▶ Avoid "water resources" / poorly constituted feeds.

▶ High level hygiene/cleanliness is advised to avoid diseases.

▶ Myth#36: Breast milk as eye drops/gutt

▶ Truth#36: Breast milk is poisonous to the eyes of babies and should not be used as gutt. It can badly damage the eye and cause chemical conjunctivitis.

▶ Myth#37: Nospamin for all forms of newborn colics.

▶ Truth#37: Most abdominal colics in newborn are from poor feeding techniques. Ensure child is not swallowing air while feeding. When wrongly use without the right indication, Nospamin causes constipation.

▶ Myth#38: Sex-starved men produce male babies.

▶ Truth#38: You cannot control the sex of your baby. Not even starving your spouse can help achieve a concentrated Y-chromosome. Remember the God factor always.

▶ Myth#39: Traditional ways of stopping convulsion.

▶ Truth#39: Setting fire, putting spoon or urinating into the mouth of a convulsing child is wrong practice. It will cause more harm. Jamming their teeth will not kill. Treat fever promptly before convulsion sets in. Take child to a hospital after convulsing episode for assessment.

▶ PREVENTION IS BETTER THAN CURE.

▶ Myth#40: Concerning reading with poor light and using glasses belonging to another.

▶ Truth#40: Reading with poor lighting, wearing another person's medicated glasses, or sitting close to the TV will not make one develop eye problems nor affect the eyes permanently. Eye muscles can only get strained or tired.

▶ PS: Looking directly at sunlight or laser light can damage your eyes.

▶ Myth#41: Eating chocolates and fried foods will give you acne commonly called pimples.

▶ Truth#41: Yes, it may be healthier to avoid excess sweets and fried foods, but it will not improve your skin as current medical knowledge, gives no support for a relationship between food and acne.

▶ Myth#42: Don't eat this or that, it will make your baby sick! E.g. Eating of snails during pregnancy is not the cause child drooling saliva like an imbecile. Eggs, sugarcane, mango, etc-makes baby sick, causes jaundice in the mother, routine drugs make babies big and labour difficult, etc

▶ Truth#42: Eating eggs, snails, etc is safe and nutritious as long as it is well cooked. Routine drugs are not directly responsible for child's weight. They help prevent and treat anaemia in pregnancy.

▶ Myth#43: Not bathing baby immediately after birth makes baby develop body odour.

▶ Truth#43: A new born should not be bathed until 6hours after birth so that it can regulate body temperature and stay warm. Early or late bathing has nothing to do with body odour.

▶ Myth#44: First milk after delivery called yellow milk is dirty and not good for the baby. It should be squeezed out to commence breast feeding after 3days of delivery.

▶ Truth#44: Colostrum, the yellow, thick breast milk just after birth is very rich in nutrients and antibodies for child's protection.

▶ Myth#45: sweet fruits like oranges, pineapple, banana, are bad for you because it contains too much sugar.

▶ Truth#45: sugar in fruits is fructose which breaks down in liver without spiking insulin levels unlike glucose. More so, fruit is high in fibre, which slows down digestion, keeping you fuller and more satisfied for long. Moderation is of essence though.

▶ Myth#46: you should poop at least once a day.

▶ Truth#46: Regular bowel movement prevents discomfort and constipation, but a perfectly healthy person may not move bowels every day. Constipation is defined as having fewer than three stools per week.

▶ Myth#47: Cold weather makes you sick.

▶ Truth#47: It may be that cold weather keeps people indoors, where germs are more likely to catch up with them from poor personal hygiene.

▶ Myth#48: men with big feet have bigger penises.

▶ Truth#48: Despite similar genetic controls for these protuberances, men with big feet do not necessarily have bigger penises. Various studies in the past have disproved this.

▶ Myth#49: All fever should be treated as malaria first!

▶ Truth#49: there are various physiological and pathological reasons for fever ranging from dehydration, hunger, stress to endocrine disorders, flu and other viral infections, to mention a few. Be sure to study the fever pattern and investigate before administering antimalarial.

GENERAL ADVICE OVER OTHER HEALTH ISSUES.

▶ Be wary of food labeled "low cholesterol". Check nutrition label, if high in saturated fat, it can raise your LDL(bad) cholesterol. Eat food low in saturated with no trans fat.

▶ Also check the serving size as you will get more cholesterol than you realized if you eat more than the serving size.

▶ Offal and organs meat such as liver, kidney are higher, in cholesterol than other cuts of meat.

Note: beef liver is high in iron, feel free to enjoy it once in a while.

▶ Food labeled "low fat" solely is not better for weight loss but its total kilojoules should be considered too.

▶ Psychiatry disorders start subtly with some forms of hallucination, mood disorders, depression etc before wandering + violence with torn clothes in public places. All forms are medically controllable. Nip in the bud.

▶ Pawpaw seeds whether dried, powdered or liquid form, contain chemicals like papain, benzylglucosinolase-antihelminthic as mebendazole for animals eg. Sheep not humans. Benefit is still poorly defined in humans.

▶ Avoid drug abuse. It causes increased rate of resistance when it is eventually needed.

▶ Food supplements are mostly less effective than fresh fruits & vegetables

▶ Beware of evil machine that scans your entire body without taking blood/urine samples to detect problems or project/prophesy ailments.

▶ It is unsafe to lick a wound or apply saliva because the mouth- "dirtiest part of the body", is full of bacteria. Stop putting yourself at the risk of infection.

▶ It is more important to maintain hydration by drinking lots of fluid. You can safely disregard the "8-glasses of water a day" rule if you eat properly and drink when you are thirsty. Moderation is the key.

▶ DESCRIPTION

ISBN-13: 978-1523890194 (CreateSpace-Assigned)

ISBN-10: 1523890193

BISAC: Health & Fitness / Health Care Issues

Health myths and facts is full of enlightening facts that will debunk some of the most perennial misconceptions we believe about our health ranging from, "toilet infection", preventing children from drinking cold water, "malaria & typhoid syndrome" and lots more, that will surprise you.

Medical practice in Nigeria and other part of Africa coupled with interactions with colleagues in diasporas have instigated the need to shed more light to the medical misconceptions, people still believe about their health that are just wrong.

It's a fun read and chances are that you will stumble across several medical myths you have always believed.

It's time to burst these myths.

▶ AUTHOR BIO

Dr. Augusta McAngus, Medical Director of SYMX Hospital Ltd. holds a degree in MB. BS from University of Benin, Nigeria and committed to community healthcare delivery in FCT, Abuja where she lives with her husband and children.

#CreateSpace eStore:
https://www.createspace.com/5983760